Living with a Disability

Living with a Disability

Cerebral Palsy, Parkinson, Epilepsy

Rachel Starr

authorHOUSE®

AuthorHouse™
1663 Liberty Drive
Bloomington, IN 47403
www.authorhouse.com
Phone: 1-800-839-8640

Published by AuthorHouse   11/19/2012

ISBN: 978-1-4772-5681-7 (sc)
ISBN: 978-1-4772-5682-4 (e)

Contents

LIVING WITH CEREBRAL PALSY

The Brown family moved to Granite Hills, Montana. The family moved there because Karen's dad lost his job as a coal miner, he found a job as a granite miner. There was a mine just outside of the city. Her dad didn't know much about granite mining but he mentioned that he was a coal miner. The foreman said, "Robert, I know you don't have any experience in granite mining but you will catch on fast, I have faith in you and you will do fine."

Granite Hills was a fairly big town the population was 30,000 the town had shops and a huge shopping center, and several churches, a bowling alley, movie theatre.

Karen was 10 years old, Karen asked, "Mom why am I different from all the other children"? Mom said, "What do you mean by different?"

Karen said, "Well the kids at school tease me and make fun of me I always sit on the steps at recess because with having braces, I can't play ball or jump rope or anything the other kids do."

Karen continues by saying, "I would cry myself to sleep because I don't like to be teased and made fun of. I asked them not to tease me; they just laughed and continued to tease and to quit acting like a baby.

Mom said, "Karen I was hoping to wait a little longer with telling you what happened when you were born. I was in labor along time. You were too big to pass through and the doctors tried everything. The doctors even tried to use forceps' in doing this the doctor hit the left temple. The doctor ended up doing a C-section but the damage was already done. This affected the right side of your body. That is why you can't use your right arm and need braces to walk."

Karen told her mom, "I also blamed God making me this way; I just wanted everything to go away and make me a whole person. I felt that I wasn't a whole person because I was damaged goods."

Mom said, "I didn't know that, why didn't you tell me?"

Karen told her, "I didn't want to say anything because I felt that you would tell me that I was being silly and not to worry about it."

Mom responded, "I'm sorry you feel that way, I would never tell you that and neither will you're dad.

Karen also said, "Mom why do you treat me different than my brothers. That really hurt. I felt you loved them more than me.?"

Mom said, "I didn't realize that I was doing that, I'm just trying to protect you so you don't get hurt. I didn't realize that you blamed God?"

Mom said, "I love you just as much as your brothers?"

Karen asked, "What is Cerebral Palsy?" Her mom said, "Cerebral Palsy is a brain injury, the injury can happen before birth, during birth or after birth."

Karen asked, "Why do some people get it and some don't?"

Mom said, "I can't answer that because I don't know the answer, it can be caused by lack of oxygen, poor head position, premature births just to name a few. Even though dad and I love you we were talking and we think that you should start going to summer camp the camp is for children with disabilities."

Karen said, "I don't want to go to any summer camp?" Mom said, "We think that you should go because we think that it would be good experience for you to be with other children with disabilities." Mom continued, "Try it for one summer and if you don't like it than you don't have to go next summer."

Karen asked, "Where is this camp?" mom said, "The camp is in a small town about 30 miles from here."

Karen thought about it, and then she said, "O.K. I'll go but I am not too thrilled about it."

When Karen got to the camp she saw two girls talking, she walked over to them and introduced herself, hi my name is Karen and I have Cerebral

Palsy." One girl said, hi my name is Susie. Susie said, "I also have Cerebral Palsy too. My mom lived on the streets and was on drugs, than she found out she was pregnant. She told me that she didn't want to keep me she wanted an abortion." But some of her friends told her about a half-way house for unwed mothers. They talked her into going and my mom stayed there until I was born." Susie continued, "I prayed to God, why am I this way?"

Karen said, "I used to ask God that too."

The other girl said, "My name is Carla, when I was about 7 I was in the back seat and a car came out of nowhere and ran into the backend of our car, and I was pinned under the front seat, the firemen had to use the Jaws of Life to get me out."

Karen asked, "I'm sorry to hear that." "What kinds of things do you do here like activities?" Susie said, "We sit around the camp fire and roast marshmallows and tell stories, sings songs."

Carla said, "Every summer the counselors talk to the Make a Wish Foundation and we go on an outing. "What kind of outings?" Karen asked. Susie said, "It's different every year."

The outing that they went on this summer was they went to a place that had a wheelchair accessible hot air balloon. Karen was excited she never did anything like this before. The balloon could only hold two people three with the instructor, Susie and Karen went together. As the balloon went around the designated area Karen said, "I feel like a bird and she spread out her arms like she was flying." Susie said, "Everything looks so small everything looks like ants."

The instructor said, "One summer we had a little boy that he was an astronaut and the balloon was a rocket ship." Karen and Susie laughed at that. After everyone had a turn the next stop was a farm that was designed for disabilities. The farm workers took the campers on a hayride those in wheelchairs were wheeled up to the wagon and then was carried onto the hay bales. They took a tour of the farm; they went by the horse stables. Susie asked, "Can we go riding?" the farm hand said, "Yes for those who want to ride."

Karen, Susie and Carla went horseback riding they were allowed to go on their own if they stayed in the secured area. Since Susie and Karen were wearing braces they only needed a leg up. Carla was in a wheel chair so she needed someone to lift her out of the wheelchair onto the horse. Karen asked, Have either of you been horseback riding before?" Susie said, "Yes," and Carla said, "No." Karen said, "She hadn't either."

The summer was almost over so it was time to go back home, the girls hugged each other and promised to write. When Karen got home she couldn't stop talking about how much fun she had.

Karen went to a school for children with disabilities when she got to middle school. Because of the teasing that occurred in the early years. Karen liked the school she made friend's right away she made friends with Jackie and her twin brother James. They both were in wheelchairs, Karen told them her story and Jackie said, "Our mom had complications and we were born too early".

Karen said, "Mom told me about multiple births, but I didn't know anyone that happened too." By 8th grade James had started to have feelings for Karen. James asked her, "Karen do you want to the soda shop sometime for a soda, we will be going to high school next year and I wanted to know will you be my girlfriend and maybe we could go steady."

Karen was surprised, she said, "James I think we are little bit too young to be thinking about that. I know I am too young and I have my whole life ahead of me, I am not ready to be serious about anyone yet." James was hurt but he said, "I understand,"

When Karen was in High school she was still was wearing braces but it was getting harder to walk. She went to the doctor and the doctor said, Karen I see that you are having trouble walking, I think we need to think of getting you a motorized scooter to help you get around a lot easier."

Karen agreed, "When will I get the scooter?" The doctor told her, "I can get the paper work done right now. You should have the scooter within a couple of weeks."

Karen loved her scooter she could go anywhere she wanted to go. One day Karen told her mom that she wanted to get her own apartment and start living on her own.

Her mom asked, "Why do you want to do that, aren't you happy here?"

Karen said, "Yes I am but I want to be more independent, and I want to eventually go to college."

Her mom said, "I don't know, I think we should talk to your father about this. I want to get his opinion."

Karen moved into her own apartment and it was not far from home so Karen could come over and mom could also come over whenever Karen needed something. Karen loved her apartment and the people that were her neighbors.

She loved to cook; she wasn't very good because her mom did all the cooking at home. At the apartment she met other people that had disabilities too. Everyone had different types of disabilities.

After Karen was on her own for a while, her mom asked, "Karen do you like living here, I didn't think you could do it?"

Mom continued, "Dad and I are very proud of you."

Karen said, "Yes I am very happy here, I'm glad I moved here. I found a job too working in a pet shop?"

Mom asked, "What will you be doing at the shop?" Karen said, "I will be working the cash register and helping with feeding the animals."

That's wonderful dear; I know you will do fine. You always loved animals." Her mom told her.

Karen said, "At first the owner was sure if he was going to hire me or not. I told him that he didn't have to worry. I may have a disability but I am very reliable and I won't let you down.

Mom said, "What did the owner say when you told him that?" Karen said, "He would give me a try and see how it works out."

The job worked out Karen was there almost a year. Karen's boss was very pleased with her work. One day her boss asked her to come into the office. Her boss said, "I have been thinking of hiring more people with disabilities, do you have anyone in mind that is looking for a job?"

Karen said, "Yes, my friend Jackie, we have been friends since High School and Susie since I was

10 I met her in summer camp for disabled kids. They both are in wheelchairs.

Her boss said, "fine could you get in touch with them and find out if they are interested in working for me and have them call me."

Karen called them, "They were excited about the job thanks for the information we will call him right away." The girls said.

Karen said, "You're welcome, call me later and let me know what happened, O.K. We will, talk to you later." Susie said.

About a year later Karen said, "Mom I love my job but I would like to give college a try." I know it won't be easy at first but I know I can do it."

Her mom said I know you can, dad and I will help you all we can." Karen had a hard time saying goodbye to all her friends at the apartment and at work. Karen knew that she was doing the right thing. She wanted to do something more with her life than doing retail jobs all her life.

The day came Karen said goodbye to her mom, her dad drove her to the school and helped her find her room, after getting Karen settled, her dad said, "Goodbye and call us if you need anything." Karen said, "I will."

LIVING WITH PARKINSON'S DISEASE

When Karen got to the college she was overwhelmed by how big it was.

Karen was putting some of her things away when a young lady walked into the room.

"Hi my name is Pam but my friends call me peanut, what's yours?" Karen said, "Hi my name is Karen, I don't have a nickname. Why do they call you peanut?" Peanut said, "Well I always was the smallest one in school I just wasn't growing, and my friends and family started calling me peanut. No one could explain it but when I was in 7th grade I started growing and by the time I got to high school I was almost as tall as everyone else in my class, everyone was used to peanut that the name stuck. Peanut continued, "May I ask you something personal?" Karen said what you want to know." Peanut asked, what happened to you, why are you in a wheelchair. Karen said, "I was born with cerebral Palsy." I started out with braces, than when I started High School I got a motorized scooter." Peanut asked "I need to think of a nickname for you." I think you look like a kitten to me." Karen said, "Why kitten do you think I look like a cat." Peanut laughed, No you just seem shy to me that's all."

Karen asked, "What classes are you taking?" Peanut said phycology, and economics I am going for nursing, what about you." Karen said I am going to be a social worker or counselor for teens and young adults. Especially people who have some type of disability." Peanut said, "We will be in some of the classes together." Karen said, "I guess we will, I think it will be fun, and we can study together." Peanut asked, "Do you have a boyfriend?" Karen said, no?" "We have to take care of that?" Peanut said. "My boyfriend Peter's roommate's name is John, I am going to talk to Peter, and maybe we could get together Friday night for dinner and a movie." Karen said no I'm not interested in a boyfriend right now maybe never." Peanut said, "Why not." Karen told her, "Who would want me as you can see I am in a wheelchair. Peanut commented, "John won't mind, his dad is in a wheelchair."

It took Karen a few weeks to feel comfortable being alone with John. John asked, "Tell me about you, family and things like that." Karen said, "I have three brothers, Robert Jr. Thomas are older than me, they are married and have families of their own. Jimmy is in high school. Karen continued, "what about you, any family." John said, "I have two sisters no brothers. My sister's names are Judy and Sandy."

Judy and I are twins but she got married after high school, mom and dad weren't too happy. They wanted us both to go to college. John continued, "May I ask you something, I was wondering, are you a Christian?" Karen said, "yes, I am." John said, "so am I." I was also wondering if you would marry me." Karen said, "you mean now." John smiled, "no not now, I mean after college."

Karen said, I never thought about getting married because as you can see, I am in a wheelchair and I don't what anyone to feel sorry for me.

John said, "I love you for what's on the inside not the outside." John continued, Karen you are a wonderful and beautiful young lady it would make me very happy and privileged if you would be my wife."

Karen smiled, "Yes John it would be my pleasure to be your wife."

When Karen got back to the dorm Peanut was in bed, so Karen was trying to be very quiet. Peanut said, "You're back, what time is it?" Karen said, I thought you were asleep, it is a little after midnight." Peanut asked, "What did you and John talk about?" Karen said, "We talked about our families, and John asked me to marry him." Peanut said, "Sat up, what did you say?" Karen said, "John asked me to marry him." Peanut said, "Are you serious, what did you tell him." Karen said, after we graduate I would marry him."

Thanksgiving was just a few weeks away and Karen went home for the weekend. Karen called her mom, "hi mom, is it alright if I bring a friend home with me. I have someone I want you and dad to meet." "Mom said, yes its fine, is it peanut." Karen said, no, it's not, my friends name is John." "Mom said, whose John." Karen said, "John is my boyfriend and before you ask, John is a Christian, can I bring him home?" "Mom said, you may, bring John." At Christmas John took Karen home to meet his family, John's family loved Karen and Karen's family loved

John. Everyone thought they would be a good match.

After graduation John and Karen got married. It was a beautiful day except for one thing. At the reception Robert lost his balance and fell into the table. Karen saw what happened. Karen said, "Dad are you alright." Dad said, "I'm fine, I just lost my balance. I have been losing my balance a lot lately." Karen said, "What's wrong." Dad said I am in the early stages of Parkinson's disease." Karen said, why you didn't tell us." Dad said, "Mom and I were going to tell you and your brothers, but we didn't want to ruin your special day." Karen said, "I know some things about Parkinson's disease, but not much." Dad said some of the symptoms are losing your balance, depression, muscle aches and pains." Dad continued, "Eventually I will be in a wheel chair." Karen asked, is there any treatment or cure." Dad said, "There is no cure, but medication will control the symptoms."

Karen and John didn't go on a honey moon because they both had to work. John said, "When we have more time we will go somewhere special just the two of us." John and Karen found a wheelchair acceptable house.

Karen wanted a baby because she loved kids. The doctor said, "Karen it is possible but I would be very careful." The doctor also made a comment, if you do have a baby I would suggest to take the baby early. I think it would be easier on you."

A few months later Karen found out she was going to have a baby. She couldn't wait to tell John.

Karen made a special supper that night. When John came home, He said, "Hi honey, Karen said, "John I have some news for you." John said, "What would that be." Karen said, "I am going to have a baby." John said, "Are you sure?" Karen said "Yes."

The big day came Karen gave birth to their son, they named him Joshua Robert after Karen's dad. Everyone came to see the baby, when Karen got home. Joshua was a happy and healthy little boy. Karen's mom said she would come over and help Karen while John was work. A couple of years later Karen had another baby, a girl this time. They named her Kimberly Jo. Again everyone came to see the baby, except Karen's dad he had to go to a nursing home, because he was going downhill fast, and mom said I can't take care of him anymore."

Karen's dad was in a wheelchair by this time. He was very depressed and he told everyone that he didn't what to live anymore. Karen and John went to the nursing home to visit. Karen said, "Dad, mom told us what you told her the other day. Why did you tell her that?" Her dad said, "I don't want to be a burden to anyone. I don't want to have anyone see me just wither up and die.

Karen said, dad you aren't a burden, we love you and we want you to be with us a long time."

A few years went by, John said, "Karen we never had a real vacation. "The kids were growing up fast and we should take them some place special. Where would you like to go?" Karen asked. John thought about it. John said, "How about we take them to Disney World." John told the kids at Christmas time that next summer they were all going on a trip. Kim said, "Dad where are we going, please tell us." John said, "If I told you it wouldn't be a surprise would it. You need to wait until it's closer to summer." Both children said, "O.K." we can't wait." A few weeks before the family were about to leave, John said, we are all going to Disney World." When they got there they saw Mickey, Minnie and all characters. When the family got there the children wanted to go on the rides. Karen couldn't go on the rides so she watched the kids and John go on the rides. After the rides they went to the Epcot Center. The children wanted to go on the boat slide. They went to the top and splashed down the waterfall. Karen wanted to go on the boat ride to but she didn't know how to achieve the situation with being in a power chair.

John said, "Karen I have an idea if you're up to it. Karen said, "What do you have in mind. John answered, "Well, I could pick you up and carry you and put you in the boat. If you want me too.

Karen told John, "Yes, I want to go." John and his family had so much fun. The weather was so hot that they enjoyed getting wet. After the rides they all went to see the shows at the theater.

There were so many to pick from they couldn't decide which one to go too.

Later that evening they went to have dinner, than went back to the hotel, they had a big day planned the next day. The next day there was a parade there were dancers and singers, they were singing, it's a small world after all. The next thing they knew the whole family were in the parade. After the parade, Mickey said, "there is a party and the whole Disney family would like to give you all a special invitation to join us." Joshua and Kim said, "Can we go PLEASE! John looked at them and said, "Yes we can." There was so much food and they all got their pictures taken with the whole gang.

It was finally time to go home, the children didn't want to go, but they couldn't wait to tell their friends about their trip. When they got home, the children asked, "Can we call grandma so we can give her the gifts we brought."

Karen said, "yes, but after we unpack and have dinner." Grandma came over and the children told her everything they did and what they saw. Karen said, "Mom how is dad doing, I haven't talked to him in a while." Mom said, He's not doing well at all, it's seems like he's depressed and confused all the time. He is in so much pain and the medication is not working and the doctors change the medication and it still doesn't work.

Karen said, "Why do you think the medication is not working." Mom said, "I'm not sure, but I think it's because he is just giving up he doesn't want to live anymore. He is going downhill so fast. I am so worried about him." Karen said, "So am I, I think tomorrow I will go and visit him.

The next day Karen's mom called Karen, "Karen I just got a call from the Nurse's at the home.

Karen asked, "What did they have to say? "The nurse told me that her father has given up and he left the planet during the night. He was in so much pain and he didn't want to live anymore.

Karen said, did you call Robert, Thomas and Jimmy yet?" Mom said, "Not yet, I wanted to call you first, since you said you were going to visit."

There was a huge turnout for the funeral. It seemed that people were coming out of the woodwork. The family saw people they haven't seen them in years.

After the funeral Karen's mom asked, Karen I just can't live in that big house anymore. I know you have a guest house. Could you ask John if I could live there, that way I can be close to family and I can be there to help you with things around the house, while John is at work?

Karen told her, I will ask John but I am sure he won't mind."

Several years went by, the children were all grown up Joshua was married about a year to a lovely girl named Nancy. They had no children yet, but a baby was on the way. Kim wasn't married yet but she had a boyfriend Sam. Karen knew that they would be hearing the sound of wedding bells soon.

LIVING WITH EPILEPSY

Kim had been dating Sam for several months now. One day Sam and Kim went driving, Kim said, "Where are we going, you said we were going to the restaurant?" Sam said, I know we will soon but I want to talk about something very important first." Kim said, Talk about what." Sam went a few feet and pulled over to the side of the road. Kim said, "What are you doing?" Sam said, "Kim I love you very much and I want to spend the rest of life with you." Kim said, "What are talking about." Sam said, "Will you have the pleasure of marrying me, pretty lady." Kim smiled, "Yes, I will." When Kim got home Kim said, "Mom something wonderful just happened, Sam asked me to marry him, I said yes."

Mom said, "We already know all about it, Sam came over a few weeks ago and talked to us. He asked dad for permission." Mom said, "Dad and I are very happy for you and Sam. Kim had invited

Sam over for dinner Saturday night to talk over the wedding plans along with her parents.

The big day came; Kim and Sam had a big wedding with all the trimmings. Kim wore her Grandmothers wedding dress, Karen also wore it. After the wedding Sam and Kim went to Washington D.C. on their honeymoon. It was late when they got in so they went to eat at the hotel dining room. The next day they took a capitol city bike tour around the city. Either one of them were on a bike in several years, Kim said, "I think the last time I was on a bike I was a child. When I started driving I stopped riding, I am totally out of shape." Sam said, I was thinking the same thing. When we get back home I think we should take up bike riding again.

After lunch they went to the planetarium at the IMAX theater, they never seen the constellations and the other stars in the daytime before. When nightfall came, Sam said, "I would like to go on another sightseeing tour. I think I would like to take the double decker tour bus though." Kim said, I would like that."

When Sam and Kim got home they went house shopping, they found a nice two story home just a few blocks away from Karen and John. About a year had gone by and Kim had made a special dinner for Sam his favorite meal, cinnamon chicken and mashed potatoes. When Sam came home he walked into the kitchen, "Sam said, hi honey I'm home." Kim said, "You're home early." Sam said, it's not early." Kim said, "I guess not, I wasn't paying attention to the time." Sam said, you have been very distracted lately, is something wrong." Kim said, "no," I have some news for you" Sam said, "what would that be." Kim said, "I am going to have a baby." Sam said, "Are you sure." Kim said, "Yes,"

A few months later Kim found out that she was going to have twins. Twins didn't run in the family so everyone was excited. Kim had given birth to, two beautiful girls. They named them Mary Jo and Margaret Ann. They all were living a very happy life, but when the girls were two years old Kim noticed changes in the girl's behavior, the girl's started twitching and have black outs, Kim called her mom, "mom something is wrong with Mary and Margaret," Karen said, "What happened." Kim told her what was happening. Karen said, "I will be right over and take you to the doctor, you are in no shape to drive."

When they arrived the doctor did several tests, the doctor came out. The doctor said, "The girls have epilepsy." Kim asked, "What is that." The doctor explained, "When you have a seizure the normal orderly pattern of electricity, when a seizure recur without a direct trigger, such as a fever the condition is called epilepsy. If a person who has both cerebral palsy and epilepsy this disruption may spread throughout the brain and cause varied symptoms all over the body.

Kim asked, "What causes epilepsy." The doctor said, "One cause is an imbalance of chemicals and body fluids, no one really knows what the cause is only what the symptoms are. I can give you medication to control the seizures." "Thank you doctor," Kim said. The doctor said, "You're Welcome and I will get the medication ready for you and some information on where you can the helmets to wear when there older, they may need them and maybe not.

When Sam got home from work Kim told him everything the doctor said. Sam said we will need to take one day at a time, and pray for strength and guidance.

When the girls started school Sam and Kim had a meeting with the teachers and the principal about the seizures we don't want to be alarmed if they start staring into space.

Mary is calmer but sometimes Margaret has more problems."

The teacher's asked, "What kind of problems?" Sam mentioned, "Sometimes when Margaret has a seizure she sometimes starts shaking and makes a fist and makes a face, like she is really mad at someone.

The teacher's said, "I don't know if we will be able to keep Margaret in school. Some of the children may not understand. The teacher looked at the principal, "What do you think?"

The principal said we appreciate for informing us, we will keep a close watch on both girls. Both girls will be accepted. If we see a problem we will contact you at a later date."

Once the girls got into middle school everything changed.

Kim called her mom, "mom the school called we have to take the girls out of school, the teachers said that the girls are not doing well in school, they can't handle their problems."

Karen said, "What do they want you to do." Kim said, they said we can home school them, I don't know anything about that." Kim said, I don't know anything about it either, but I can go on the internet and see what I can find." Kim said, "O.k. talk soon" A couple of days later Karen called back. "Kim I have some information for you" Kim said, "what did you find out."

Karen said, "There are seven steps you need to take."

- You need to find out about what the laws are because they are different in each state
- Contact a local homeschool support groups, so you can organize field trips, spelling bees with other home school families
- Subscribe to a homeschooling magazine where you can find various subjects and different learning methods
- Choose subjects and books for the girls
- Set up an area in your home to keep your supplies
- Design a routine for the girls so they know what subjects they will be doing and what time of day they will have that subject
- Stay focused and have fun

Kim said, "That is a lot of things to remember." Karen said, "I know, just pray every day and you will be fine."

Kim called the school, the school said that there were some forms to fill out, and when the school received that the books and supplies would be sent out. When the supplies arrived Kim said, "On Monday, Wednesday, and Friday morning we will be doing math, science, and reading. In the afternoon we will have history, and social studies. On Tuesday and Thursday morning we will have a foreign language class. And in the afternoon we will have art. The girls looked at their mom, Mary said, "Why a foreign language."

Kim said, Depending on your grades at the end of the year your dad and I will take you to that country that you choose for a vacation. The girls picked France; Kim bought a cd/dvd combination on France and learn the French language.

Mary and Margaret practiced there French on their dad when he got home from work. After dinner they sat down as a family to watch the DVD so they could pick out what they wanted to see.

The day arrived, they were very tired when they when they got to Paris. They all went to the hotel and after they rested they went out to dinner. They had dinner inside the Eiffel Tower; mom had to make reservations at least two weeks ahead of time. The restaurant was very popular and very busy. After dinner they all went shopping at some of the small shops and got Ice Cream. Later that night, they went to see a light projection show at the Eiffel tower the guide told them about observation tower. The guide said, "the elevator was 59 feet to the top, and then the guide told them that nighttime was the best time to go to the top. Every hour from nightfall to 2:00 in the morning there are bursts of shimmering display of light. The beams of light shoot upward through the tower structure." The guide also said, "That there were 335 projectors spilling through the tower." Mary and Margaret liked the show, they both said, "It's like Christmas and 4th of July rolled into one big package.

After a good night's sleep they were on the go again, the girls had their camera's ready they went to the different museums and art galleries. They also went on a boat ride down one of the local rivers, to see the sights and then at night they went on a dinner cruise, and boat tour seeing the water glowing in moonlight. The next day they all went to Disneyland, there was a parade with several floats. While they saw a stuntman show and they took a ride behind the props. They also saw an Indiana Jones show and after the show they got special invitation to see how the movie was made and got to meet the actors.

The vacation was over and Sam had to go back to work and school would be starting soon. Mary and Margaret had taken a lot of pictures and asked, "Mom can we make a scrapbook of our trip in art class." Kim said, yes, that would be a good idea."

When everyone got home they stopped and picked up something for dinner and then unpacked. Kim called her mom, "mom I thought I would let you know that were home." Karen said, "Kim I am so glad your home, I didn't want to call while you were on vacation." Kim said, "What wrong," Karen said, "your dad had a heart attack," Kim said, "Is he alright." Karen said, "He's fine he just needs to take it easy for a while, I just checked on him and he was sleeping." Kim said, "the girls have presents for you both, would it be alright if we come over for a while." Karen said, "Yes, I want to hear all about your trip."

When they arrived John was up, the girls said, grandpa are you o.k. John said, "I'm fine I am just tired and I have to take everything a lot slower, and I thank God that it wasn't too serious."

Kim said I'm glad your o.k. we don't want to lose you, and we all love you and mom." John said, "Thank you honey I love all of you too."

With John still recovering from his heart attack, Karen needed more help around the house. Some of the things John helped her with like laundry and some of the household chores. Kim came over a couple times a week after school to help out.

A few years later John couldn't take care of Karen any more they were both getting older and he couldn't take care of her. John decided to put Karen in an Assisted Living Facility with a nursing home close by. John knew she would get better care there. John went to visit her every day.

A few years later Kim and Sam were having dinner out with some friends; the hostess came over and told Kim that there was a phone call at the desk. Kim followed her to the entrance. Kim took the call in the lobby, the call was from Mary, Kim said, "Mary what's wrong." The nurse at the facility called and said that Grandma died. Grandpa was there when it happened. The police were here, they said that there was an accident.

The girls were informed by one of the nurses that they heard her dad say Karen I love you and I always will. But I can't live without you.

John had crashed the car on purpose so he could be with his beloved wife Karen forever in Heaven.